Design & Presented By

Calmly Productions

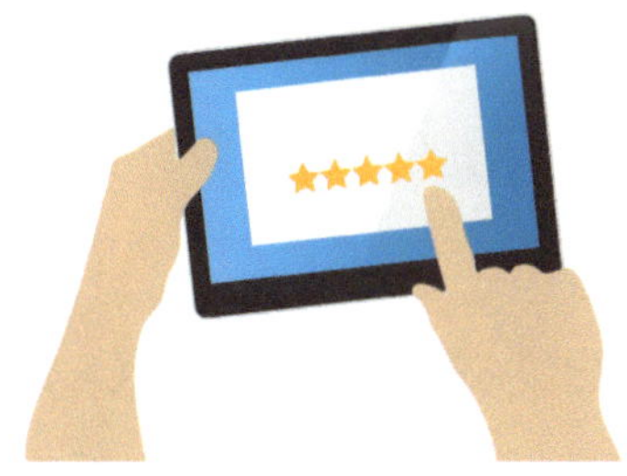

If you enjoyed this book, please consider leaving a review to share your thoughts!
Thank you!

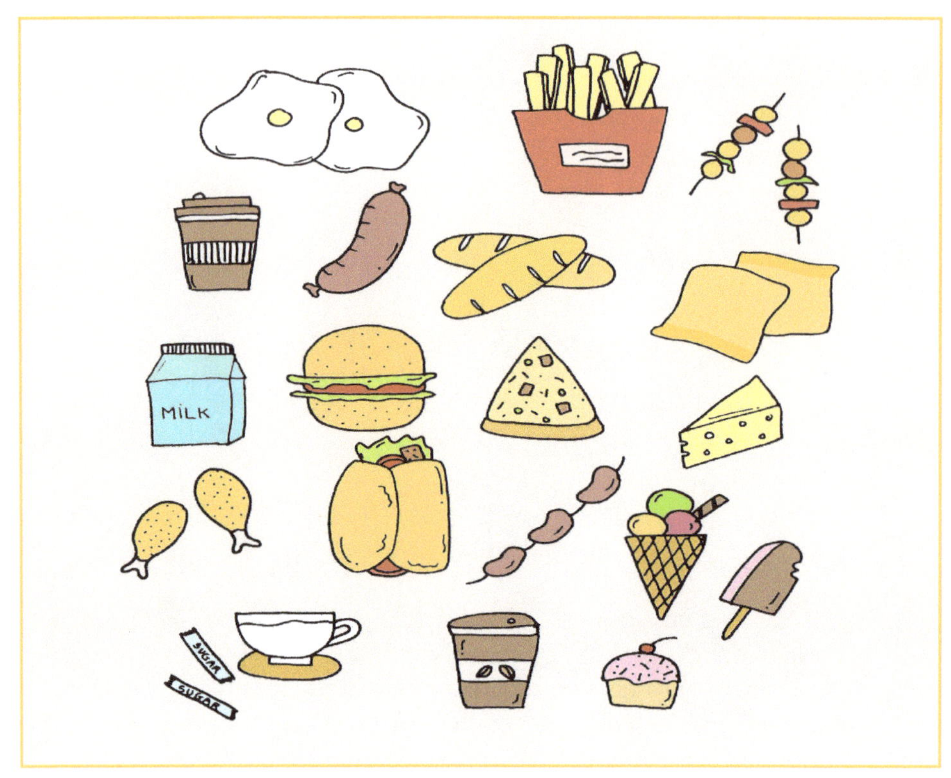

What is Junk Food?

Junk food is tasty but not very healthy. It includes things like chips, candy, cookies, and fast food. These foods have lots of sugar, salt, and unhealthy fats, but not many vitamins or nutrients. Eating too much junk food can make us feel tired and not so good. It's important to eat healthy foods like fruits, vegetables, and whole grains to stay strong and happy!

Unscramble the Words:

NCTADY __________
(Hint: It's sweet and comes in many colors)
ERUGRBE __________
(Hint: You get this at fast food places)
PHICS __________
(Hint: Crunchy and comes in a bag)
FSTA ODOF __________
(Hint: Quickly made meals)
IOKOCE __________
(Hint: Sweet treat, often with chocolate chips)
IRFTU __________
(Hint: Grows on trees and is sweet)
IKML __________
(Hint: You drink this, comes from cows)
RETWA __________
 (Hint: Keeps you hydrated)
REANIBWOR __________
(Hint: Sweet and chewy, comes in different flavors)
ZAIZP __________
(Hint: Cheesy, with toppings, often cut in slices)
SGEVIEGELATB __________
(Hint: Healthy and grows in the garden)
EKCA __________
(Hint: A sweet dessert, often with frosting)
DIASWCNH __________
(Hint: Two slices of bread with something tasty in
 the middle)

What's Good and What's Not Good Stuff:

Quick and Easy: Junk food is fast to grab and eat when you're hungry and don't have much time.

Tasty Treats: It often tastes really yummy and is super fun to eat.

Cheap and Cheerful: Sometimes junk food costs less than other foods, so it's easy to get.

Lots of Choices: There are many kinds of junk food, like chips and cookies, so you can pick your favorite.

Feel-Good Moment: Eating junk food can make you feel happy and give you a quick boost of energy.

Not-So-Good Stuff:

Not Much Nutrition: Junk food doesn't have the vitamins and minerals your body needs to grow strong and healthy.

Too Much Sugar and Fat: It has lots of sugar and fat, which isn't good for your body and can make you feel tired later.

Can Lead to Extra Weight: Eating too much junk food can make you gain weight, which isn't healthy.

Energy Ups and Downs: It can give you lots of energy at first but then make you feel tired and grumpy.

Hard to Stop Eating: Sometimes it's easy to eat too much junk food because it tastes so good, and that can be bad for you.

Homemade Burger Recipe for Kids

Ingredients:
1 lb ground turkey or chicken
1/2 cup grated carrot
1/4 cup chopped spinach or broccoli
1/4 cup whole wheat breadcrumbs
1 egg
1 tsp dried herbs (like oregano)
4 whole wheat burger buns
4 slices of cheese
Sliced tomatoes, lettuce, cucumbers
Plain yogurt (for spreading)

Instructions:

Mix: Combine ground meat, grated carrot, chopped veggies, breadcrumbs, egg, herbs, and a pinch of salt.

Shape: Form into 4 patties.

Cook: Heat a skillet over medium. Cook patties 5-6 minutes per side, until cooked through.

Toast: Lightly toast buns.

Assemble: Place patties on buns, top with cheese, veggies, and a dollop of yogurt.

Enjoy: Serve and eat!
Perfect for a fun and nutritious meal!

Circle the Junk Food

Apple

Candy

Carrot

Chips

Yogurt

Burger

Nuts

Cookie

Water

Grapes

Pizza

Celery

Soda

Nuggets

Banana

French Fries

Strawberries

Popcorn

Noodles

Cake

Kiwi

Donuts

Turkey

Ice Cream

Milkshake

Sausages

Fish

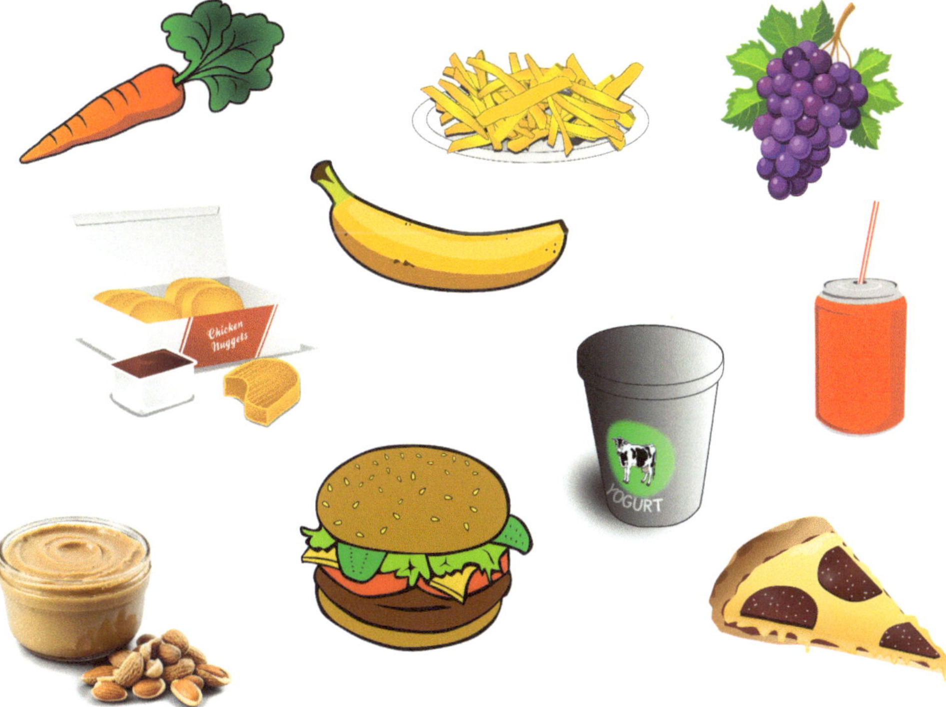

How to Control Junk Food Habit

Choose healthy snacks: pick fruits, veggies, or nuts instead of candy or chips.

Drink water: drink water or milk instead of sugary sodas and juices.

Enjoy treats occasionally: it's okay to have junk food sometimes, but not every day.

Make healthy food fun: turn fruits and veggies into fun shapes or eat them with yummy dips.

Ask for help: talk to your parents about making healthier choices together.

by making these simple changes, you can enjoy tasty foods and keep your body happy and strong!

What Happens When Junk Food Goes Into Our Body?

Quick Energy, Then a Crash: Junk food gives a fast energy boost, but soon makes you feel tired.

Sugar Attack on Teeth: Sugar in junk food invites germs that can cause painful cavities.

Sticky Fat: Junk food has fat that can slow you down and make it harder to play.

Upset Tummy: Too much junk food can make your stomach feel bad.

Brain Fog: Junk food can make it hard to think clearly and focus.

Tips for Eating Ice Cream and Candies

 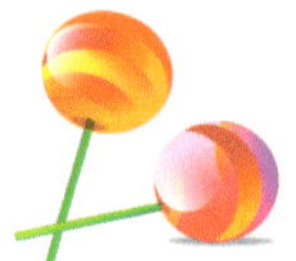

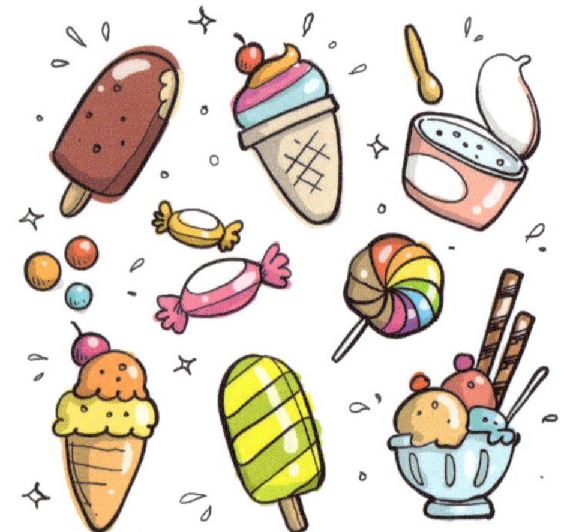

Special Treats: Enjoy them sometimes, not every day.

Small Amounts: Have just a little bit.

After Meals: Eat sweets after a healthy meal.

Brush Teeth: Brush your teeth after eating sweets.

Drink Water: Drink water to wash away the sugar.

Stay Active: Play and be active after enjoying treats.

This way, you can enjoy your treats and stay healthy!

Distinguish Healthy and Unhealthy

Write down their names in the right column

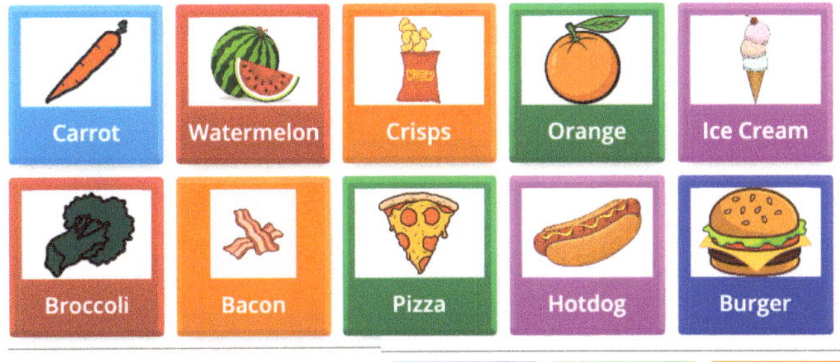

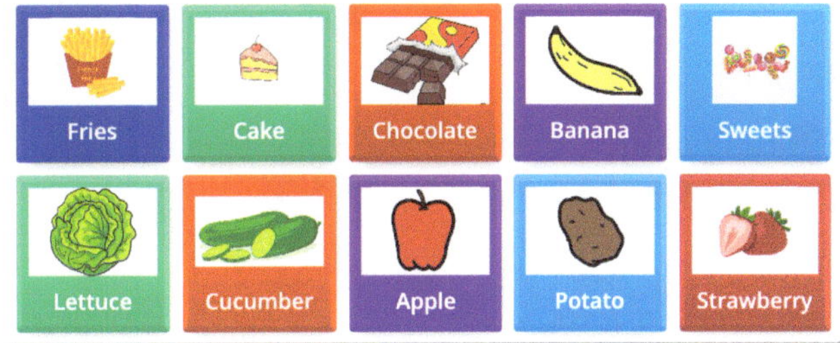

Healthy	UnHealthy

Benefits of Home Food

Full of Nutrients:
Home-cooked meals are packed with vitamins and minerals that help you grow strong and healthy.

Fresh and Tasty:
Home food uses fresh ingredients, making it delicious and full of natural flavors.

Energy Boost:
Eating home-cooked meals gives you steady energy to play, learn, and have fun all day.

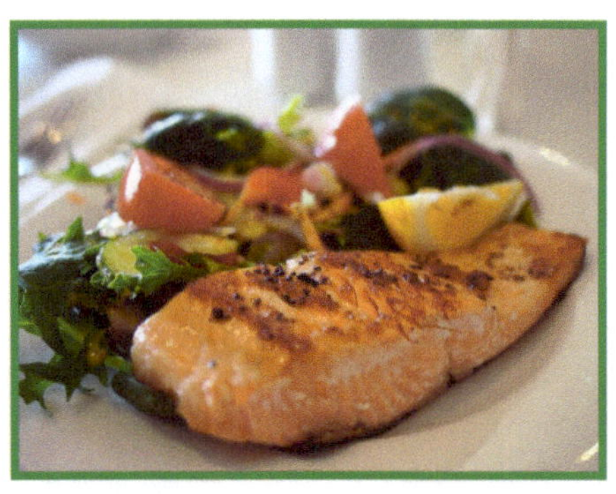

Helps You Grow:
Nutritious home food supports your growth and keeps your body strong.

Healthy Habits:
Cooking and eating at home teaches you good eating habits that can last a lifetime.

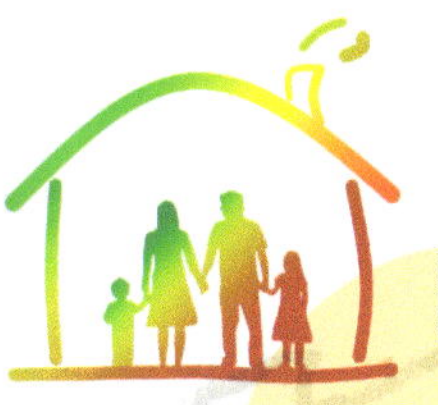

Family Time Fun!

Making and eating meals at home is like a special family adventure! You get to:

Cook Together: Be little chefs and help mix, stir, and taste.

Share Stories: Talk about your day and tell funny stories while you eat.

Try New Foods: Discover yummy, healthy foods that make you strong.

Feel Proud: Enjoy the food you made together and feel happy.

Cooking and eating with your family makes mealtime fun and helps everyone stay healthy!

Chef of the day
Write down your own healthy recipe

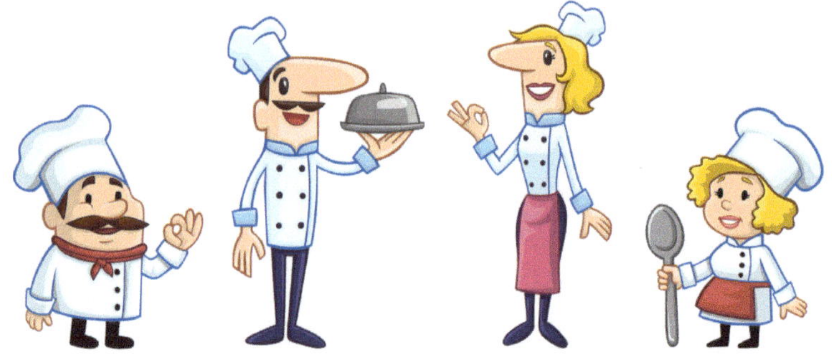

Ingredient:

____

____

Recipe:

____

____

____

____

Before we dive into the topic of obesity, it's important to understand how it happens and what it's linked to.

What is Obesity?

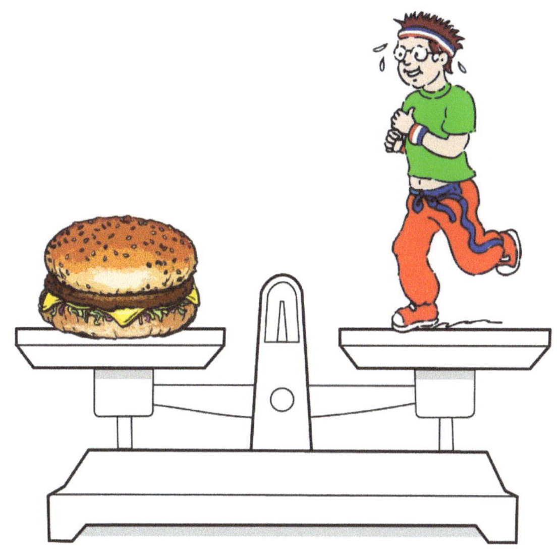

Obesity is when a person has too much body fat. This can happen when they eat more calories than their body uses, often from eating too many unhealthy foods and not being active enough. Obesity can lead to health problems and make it harder to move and play.

Here's what you need to know:

Too Much Junk Food: Eating lots of sugary, fatty foods can make you gain extra weight.

Not Enough Activity: Playing video games or watching TV a lot instead of running and playing outside can also lead to obesity.

Health Problems: Being very overweight can make it hard to run, play, and can cause health problems like feeling tired or getting sick more often.

Healthier picks

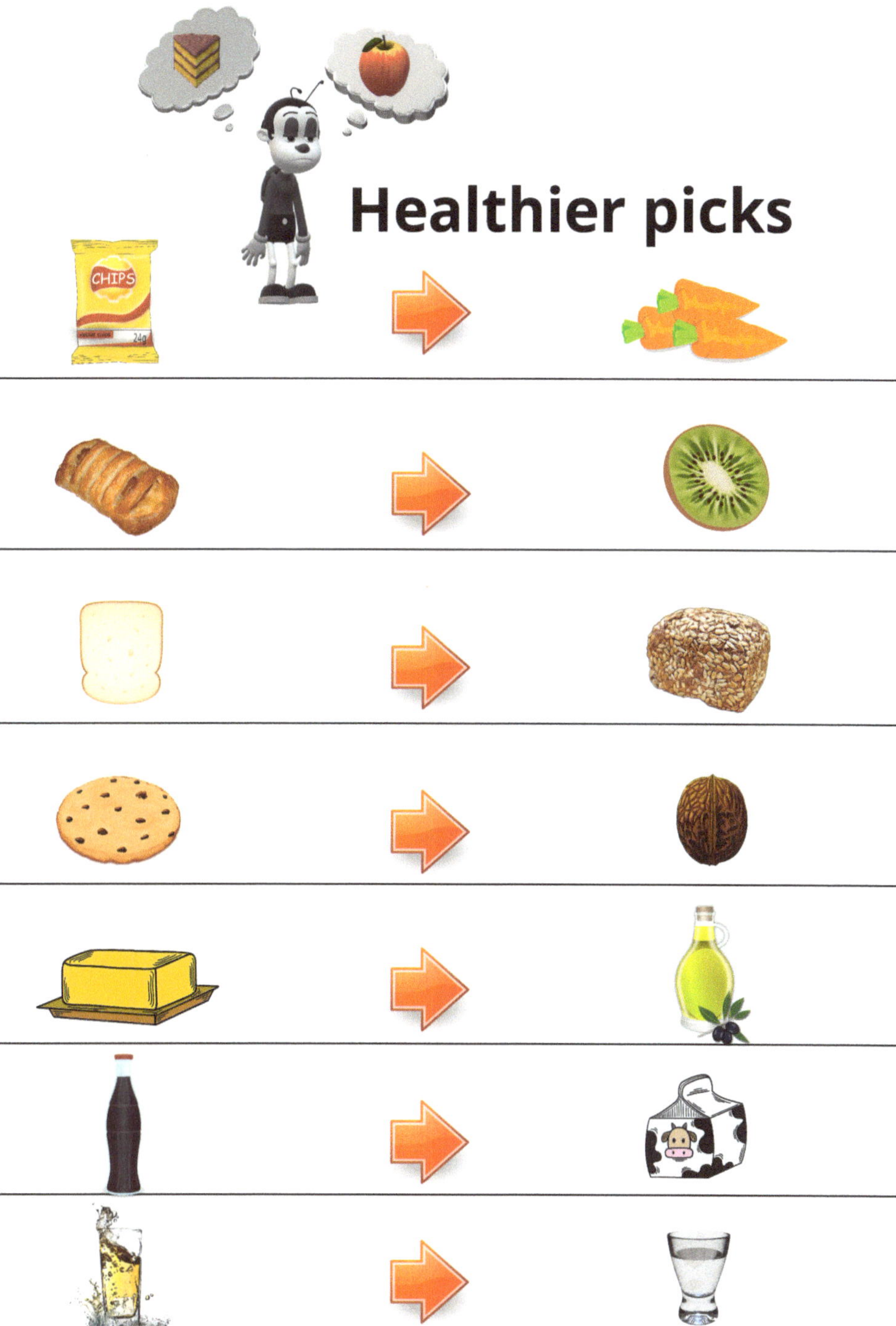

Plan ahead: There's no better way to handle cravings than planning your meals and snacks ahead of time.

Why Spicy Instant Noodles Aren't Good for You?

Spicy noodles might taste yummy, but they're not very good for your body. **Here's why:**

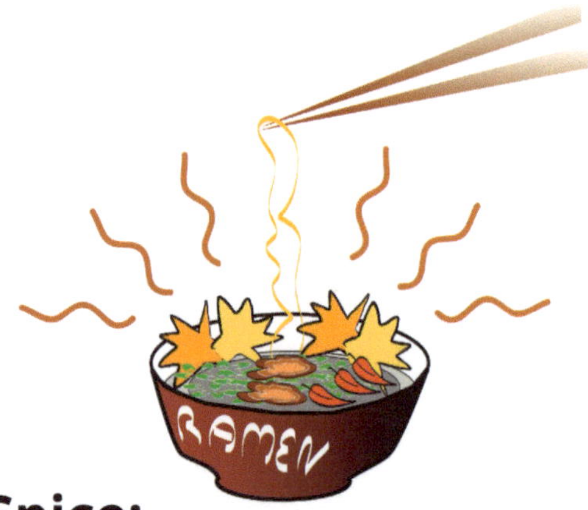

Too Much Spice:

Spicy noodles have a lot of hot spices. Eating too much spicy food can hurt your tummy and make it feel uncomfortable.

Lots of Salt:

Spicy noodles have a lot of salt. Too much salt isn't good for you and can make you feel thirsty and tired.

Harmful Ingredients:

Spicy noodles often have things like artificial flavors and preservatives. These are not natural and aren't good if you eat them a lot.

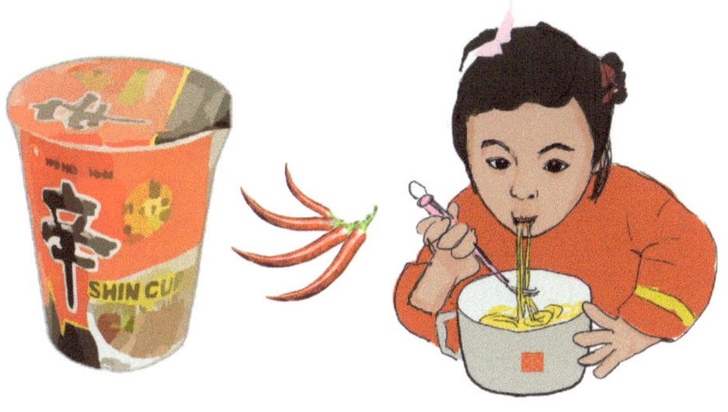

High in Calories:

Spicy noodles have a lot of calories, which can make you gain weight if you eat them too often. They don't have many vitamins or good nutrients your body needs.

Tummy Trouble:

Eating spicy noodles too much can make your tummy hurt and can even make it hard to go to the bathroom.

Conclusion:

While it's okay to have spicy noodles once in a while, eating them regularly is not a good idea. They can make your tummy hurt and don't give your body the good stuff it needs. Try to choose healthier snacks most of the time.

EASY HEALTHY PIZZA

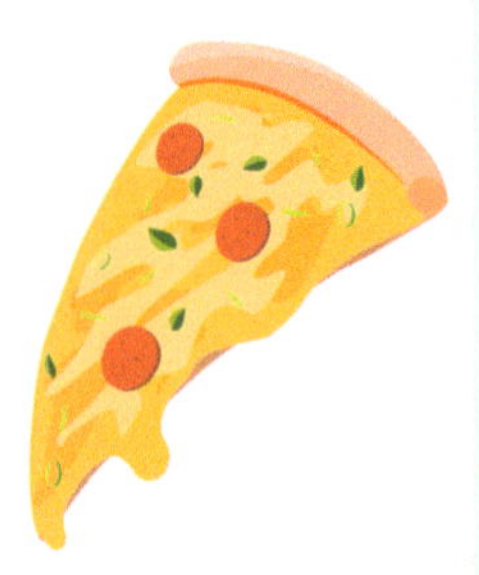

Ingredients
3 wholemeal 20 cm pita breads
¼ cup tomato paste (no added salt is best)
½ cup Chicken(optional)
½ red capsicum, thinly sliced
4 button mushrooms, thinly sliced
½ cup diced fresh or tinned pineapple
1 tomato, thinly sliced
½ cup mozzarella cheese, grated
1 handful fresh basil to garnish

Serves 2 adults (1 pizza each) and 2 children (½ pizza each)
Preparation time: 5 mins
Cooking time: 10 mins

Method
Preheat oven to 200°C (180°C fan forced).
Place bread onto oven trays and spread with tomato paste. Arrange all other ingredients over the bread. Top with cheese.
Bake in preheated oven for 10 minutes or until golden.
Remove from oven and allow to cool slightly.
Top with fresh basil. Cut into wedges and serve.

Calories Chart for Snacks

Snacks	Calories Per Serving
Gummy Bears	About 140 calories (20 pieces)
Hard Candy	About 60 calories (3 pieces)
Chocolate Candy	About 150 calories (small pack)
Potato Chips	About 150 calories (small pack)
Tortilla Chips	About 140 calories (10 chips)
Milk Chocolate Bar	About 210 calories (1 small bar)
Dark Chocolate	About 170 calories (1 small bar)
Chocolate Chip Cookies	About 160 calories (2 cookies)

Portion Size Matters: Eating a lot of any snack can add up in calories quickly.

Special Treats: Candies, chips, and chocolate are okay for special treats, but not all the time.

Write what you think about
Junk Food vs Healthy Food

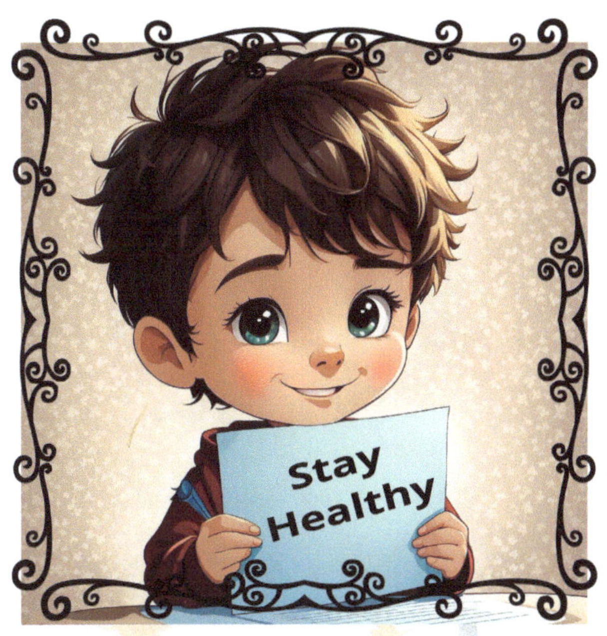

Remember, healthy choices help you feel good and have lots of energy. Eat colorful fruits and veggies, whole grains, and drink plenty of water. Enjoy treats sometimes, but mostly eat healthy foods. Play outside, limit screen time, get enough sleep, and keep clean. Enjoy meals with your family and stay connected.

Stay healthy and enjoy every moment!

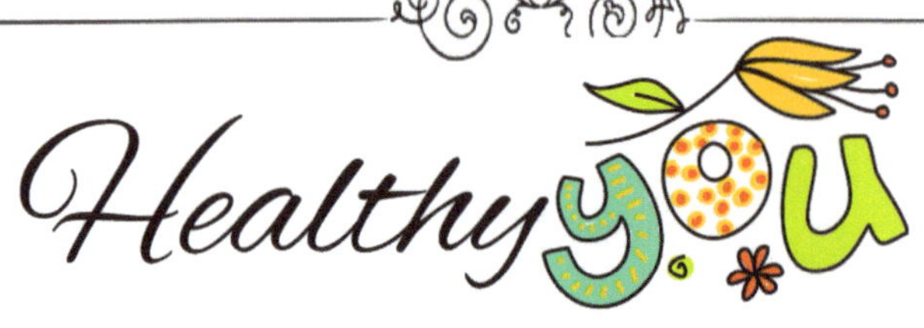

As a food expert, the writer has focused on healthy eating throughout this book, aiming to motivate kids to choose healthier options and avoid junk and fast food. The main reason for creating this book is to help you understand how important it is to eat foods that help your body grow strong and stay healthy. While junk food might seem tasty, it doesn't give your body the good stuff it needs to play, learn, and have fun. By making smart food choices, you'll have more energy, feel better, and be ready for all the exciting adventures that come your way.